Heart
of the
OR

AORN and Perioperative Nursing

The Association of periOperative Registered Nurses (AORN) is the national association committed to improving patient safety in the surgical setting. AORN is the premier resource for perioperative nurses, advancing the profession and the professional with valuable guidance as well as networking and resource-sharing opportunities. AORN promotes safe patient care and is recognized as an authority for safe operating room practices and a definitive source for information and guiding principles that support day-to-day perioperative nursing practice.

AORN Vision and Mission

Vision statement
AORN is the leader in advocating for excellence in perioperative practice and health care.

Mission statement
AORN's mission is to promote safety and optimal outcomes for patients undergoing operative and other invasive procedures by providing practice support and professional development opportunities to perioperative nurses. AORN will collaborate with professional and regulatory organizations, industry leaders, and other health care partners who support the mission.

Core Values

AORN's core values reflect what is truly important to the association:
- Communication—open, honest, collaborative
- Quality—reliable, timely, accountable
- Innovation—creative, risk taking, leading edge
- Diversity—teamwork, inclusion, respect

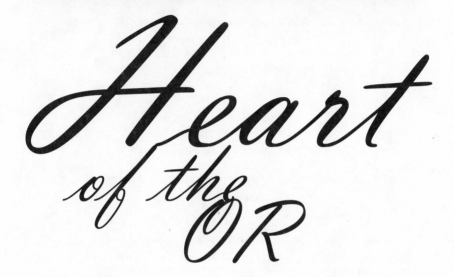

Heart of the OR

Stores of growth, discovery, and innovation
by perioperative nurses

Edited by:
Carina Stanton, MA

Preface by:
Linda Groah, RN, MSN, CNOR, NEA-BC, FAAN

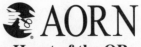

AORN
Heart of the OR
Copyright © 2011 AORN, Inc.

Director of Publishing: Liz Haigh
Editor: Carina Stanton
Associate Editor: Helen Starbuck Pashley
Copy Designers: Kurt Jones and Cathie Bigam
Director of Production: Terry Isaacs

2170 South Parker Road
Suite 400
Denver, CO 80231-5711
(800) 755-2676
(303) 755-6300
www.aorn.org

ISBN 978-1-888460-06-3   Printed in United States

Table of Contents

Table of Contents

continued

AORN thanks *Heart of the OR* contributors
for sharing their stories in this collective effort to advance
knowledge and promote patient safety.

Foreword

Storytelling is a natural part of the human condition.
We tell stories to share experiences, to share knowledge and
to teach others how to avoid mistakes and do things better.
Stories also give us a way to remember, to keep moments and
people from being lost over time.

Nurses tell great stories, whether they are explaining a
technical practice or remembering a patient, and I find that
most stories from nurses combine the two. In fact, I've found
that nurses often teach through sharing their own experiences.
And this makes sense. Learning the recommended practice for
counting sponges is part of a perioperative nurse's education,
but remembering the story of a nurse surrounded by bags
of bloodied sponges she has counted over and over again,
knowing that missing sponge is in her patient, that is what
stays in readers' minds and reminds them why they need to
follow the recommended practice.

The seed for this collection of stories began with an online
series I started in *AORN Connections* called "From the Field."
I needed an outlet to share, in their own words, the wonderful
stories perioperative nurses send me. As AORN's news editor,
I have had the opportunity to listen to so many stories from
perioperative nurses, and I have done my best to share these
stories in a way that captures the spirit of the storytellers
and the essence of their message. But there is something
important about sharing stories in the teller's own words.

The voices in this collection of stories share lessons from
the operating room. Some stories are practical innovations
for how to improve safety, some stories admit mistakes
made, and some stories remember the patients that didn't

survive but left lasting impressions. Many stories also speak to new nurses, encouraging them to stand tall, stay focused, and remember always to fight for the patient. Other stories remind seasoned nurses what they do best to mentor others and what they can do to improve their practice, not only for patients, but for the profession of perioperative nursing.

In one story, a nurse remembers the wisdom of a perioperative colleague who expects the worst of situations and the best of people. In a sense, this collection of stories does just that—it helps perioperative nurses be prepared for what can go wrong, and it encourages them to be proud they work among perioperative nurses who are committed to getting it right.

Carina Stanton
Senior News Editor, AORN
June 2010

Preface

"The Heart of the OR" – what is it? How can it be defined? I have seen it in the eyes of the novice nurse as she walks into the OR for the first time. I have witnessed it as the perioperative nurse reassures the elderly man that his wife of 50 years will be taken care of as if she was the nurse's own grandmother. I have heard it in the soft lullaby being sung by the nurse as she takes the infant from the mother's arms and enters through the double doors of the surgical suite. I have seen the heart of the OR in the hands of the nurse as she comforts and reassures the teenager before he drifts off to sleep, and I have seen it in the tears of the surgical team as they accept, in spite of all their efforts, the fate of the trauma patient who just died on the OR bed. As you read these stories, you will feel the pulse of perioperative nurses doing what they do every day to advocate for patients when they are unable to advocate for themselves, passionately caring for the surgical patient in unique and extraordinary ways.

Caring is not just what perioperative nurses do, it is who we are. Caring is demonstrated in many different ways – it is the essence of the nurse/patient relationship. Caring is not always spoken or written about and is frequently ignored or considered not valuable. Caring has been described as the essence of nursing. It is caring that enables perioperative nurses to deliver safe, quality nursing care in an environment filled with technology. Technology and caring are commonly viewed as opposite ends of the spectrum – technology reflects a mechanistic perspective, while caring reflects a humanistic perspective. We have come to depend on technology in the care of the surgical patient, and it would be difficult for us to care for patients in its absence. Perioperative nurses, however, have historically identified, embraced, and incorporated into their practice ways to promote and protect human dignity and caring as an essential partner with technology. Caring as a nursing action is a series of interactions with the patient and with other members of the surgical team. It transforms the mechanistic world of the OR into a caring environment. It preserves and promotes the human spirit. It is the heart of the OR.

Story telling has a rich history and is an important aspect of all cultures. It is used to educate and preserve a culture and to instill moral values. Stories also are used to gather and disseminate knowledge, to encourage collaboration, to generate new ideas, and to ignite change. The stories in this collection address a wide range of topics. Each story teller is motivated to protect the patient, to preserve human dignity, and to make a difference in the life of an individual as they provide care during a surgical intervention. As you read these stories I hope you will pause and reflect on the extraordinary things that you do every day that go unnoticed as you make a difference to your patients. You are the Heart of the OR.

Linda Groah, RN, MSN, CNOR, NEA-BC, FAAN
CEO and Executive Director, AORN
June 2010

Retrieving a Retained Sponge

Karen McKown, RN, BSN, CNOR, BC
Columbia, South Carolina

A s OR nurses, we are a definitive breed of nurses. We have all "been there and done that," and when it comes to surgery we know the procedures, expectations, and desired outcomes when our duties are performed according to the standards of nursing we hold so sacred.

We all have cases that we could do with our eyes shut because we are accustomed to the routine. These cases are flawless—surgical counts are correct, surgeons acknowledge staff members for "jobs well done," and our patients are off to the postanesthesia care unit (PACU) for a successful recovery, and we are ready to do it again. We feel good about ourselves as professional nurses because we contributed to the success of our patient's surgery; but we also have those days when certain cases seem to send out alarms that "this case is going to be a disaster before it has begun." As perioperative nurses, we have that intuitive insight. I had one of those experiences a few years ago that almost convinced me to give up nursing altogether. If it had not been for the support and encouragement I received from my former OR manager and the surgeon involved, I would not be the nurse I am today.

As experienced general surgery nurses, I am sure you are familiar with the abdominal-perineal resection procedure. It is a major surgery. The surgical set-up is crucial and must be performed prior to the patient's arrival to the surgical suite. The paramount focus must be establishing a correct baseline count that includes all instruments and all soft counts (eg, sponges, sutures). I cannot stress enough, however, the importance of having experienced nurses and surgical technologists that MUST communicate with each other at all times when such a critical surgery is performed.

I was the second shift relief nurse for the abdominal-perineal resection case that began around 7:30 that morning and was still underway at 3:00 p.m. when I arrived. I knew it was going to be one of those "oh no, what have I walked into" cases when I looked around the OR suite and saw all the instruments on the back tables and bags of trash lined against the walls. I saw one surgeon at the patient's abdomen working tediously and a second surgeon working at the patient's rectum. I was informed by the circulator that the instrument count was not correct because so many additional instruments had been needed throughout the day, and the instrument count sheets did not reflect what had been added to the sterile field. I completed the relief count with the second shift surgical technologist, and our soft count was correct. I was uncomfortable with the incorrect instrument count at the time of the shift change, but the general consensus in the room was that radiology personnel would take an X-ray before the surgeons closed the incisions, and both surgeons were aware of the intention to take an X-ray at the end of the case.

The case continued well into the night. When the surgeons finally began closing, I wanted to complete a soft count. I approached my surgical technologist, gloved and ready to begin counting laparotomy sponges. The technician refused to count because she stated, "we were going to get an X- ray anyway at the end of the case." She basically ignored me. I asked again to complete a count, and she reluctantly counted with me. Fortunately, our soft count was again accurate.

It was 10:30 p.m. and the patient had been on the OR bed for 15 hours. Everyone in the room was anxious to get the patient out of the OR as quickly as possible and into the PACU. The surgeons were physically and mentally exhausted. The second surgeon left to make his rounds before the final wound closure. I proceeded to count laparotomy sponges again at the end of the procedure. The surgical technologist again refused to count with me, again stating that it was a "waste of time, we were going to get an X-ray anyway."

This is where I made my first mistake. I did not insist she count with me; instead, I proceeded to count on my own. My second mistake was not informing the primary surgeon of the situation before he left the OR to talk with the patient's family. I called the X-ray technician in at the end of the case and he took X-rays of the patient's abdomen. The anesthesia care provider extubated the patient and we transferred him to PACU.

My third mistake was allowing the patient to leave the OR without confirmation from the radiologist that there were no retained sponges or instruments seen on the film; but at that time, my facility did not have a mandatory policy that required the patient remain in the OR suite until the radiologist called with his report. The radiologist who read the X-ray thought that he saw something low in the patient's abdominal cavity, but from his phone conversation with the surgeon, the object he saw was identified as the Salem sump drain. The surgeon went home. By now, it was after midnight. Everyone had gone home except me. I counted my laparotomy sponges and came up with 79. I counted again and again hoping that I would find a missing laparotomy sponge concealed in a bloody drape, towel, or glove; but it was not to be. I knew that 80th laparotomy sponge was inside my patient.

I vividly remember emptying the contents of those 14 bags of trash with bloody drapes, gowns, gloves, and tissue all on the floor. I was there alone, going through all that trash searching for one missing sponge that I never found. I knew what I had to do. Making the call to the surgeon that night was one of the hardest things I have ever done. He asked me if I had counted and I told him what had happened. He came back to the hospital a short time later, brought the patient back to the OR, and, with the patient under anesthesia, he retrieved the missing lap just under the abdominal incision. The patient required no further surgeries and recovered without incident.

The surgeon came to me later and asked why this incident happened. I knew I was totally at fault and ready to accept any punishment, reprimand, or termination. Instead of reprimanding me, this surgeon thanked me for what I had done. He said that if I had not followed through with my surgical conscience, that sponge would have remained in the patient's abdomen and the consequences could have been disastrous for the patient, the hospital, and for him.

I cannot begin to tell you how much his support and

compassion meant to me at that time. My OR manager along with risk management and department personnel within the facility worked closely together to implement policies and procedures to ensure that incidents such as this one never happen again. My OR manager continued to reassure me that I was a good nurse, and most important, a nurse with a surgical conscience that embodied integrity and honesty. She has been my mentor through the years that have followed. Today, I am a nurse educator working at a different facility. OR nursing is my passion. I would not have had the opportunities I have today if not for the support and encouragement from my former OR manager, my peers, and that incredible surgeon who looked beyond the mistake and recognized the potential.

The fear of failure, inexperience, and poor communication and interpersonal skills are potential barriers to any nurse's success. We must help nurses overcome these barriers with continued guidance, support, and encouragement from our mentors, leaders, educators and our peers. As perioperative nurses, as well as nurses in all disciplines, we have an ethical duty and responsibility to promote and maintain the integrity of nursing. Let us never forget why we became nurses and always remember the Nightingale Pledge, "I will do all in my power to maintain and elevate the standards of my profession." As surgical nurses, we hold values and beliefs that contribute to our delivery of patient care. We must always hold our surgical conscience above all else. It is what makes us a definitive breed of nurses.

Staying Calm for the Patient

Jennifer Ogden, RN, BSN, CNOR
Shawnee Mission, Kansas

I can vividly remember what it felt like to be a nursing student and finally a new graduate nurse. Being new in the operating room can be extremely intimidating and stressful, no matter how many people tell you that your mistakes are common ones, that you'll make more as you learn, and not to worry. But I did worry and I was stressed. I cried about it, and I had moments when I wondered if I had made the right career decision. I know I am not the only nurse to have felt this way.

Every perioperative nurse probably can recall a few moments when the light went on for them and some of the overwhelming amount of information they were given finally made sense. For me, one of those moments happened while I was still a nursing student completing my senior year practicum in the OR at a large university medical center. I was a nursing intern for nearly six months, and during that time I learned the basics of circulating and scrubbing for general and peripheral vascular cases.

One morning, expecting my first case of the day to be one of the typical elective general cases, my preceptor and

I arrived at report to find that a trauma patient was being taken into our room. The patient had multiple gunshot wounds to the abdomen and groin and had just arrived in the OR. We were to relieve the nurse who had worked the night shift.

At this point in my practicum, I felt relatively comfortable circulating a cholecystectomy or a breast biopsy. I had no idea how to care for a trauma patient, so I followed the lead of my preceptor. I remember that the room was filled with people doing many things: anesthesia care providers were placing IV and arterial lines, nurses were calling the blood bank for blood, nurses were opening supplies, and other individuals were counting instruments with the scrub person. It looked like an impossible mess. How did they know what to do?

I stood back and watched everyone complete their tasks. Finally, the surgeon made the incision and the surgical procedure was under way! I was curious to see how the case would progress and wanted to watch the surgeon and the residents as they explored the patient's abdomen. My preceptor, however, reminded me of what needed to be done on our end, and I quickly became engrossed with catching up on important patient documentation, organizing the room so that counts would be easier, and listening for and providing for the needs of the surgical team.

Things began to settle down as the surgeon located damaged structures and began the necessary repairs. The anesthesia care provider was beginning to get the patient stabilized, and we all felt a little more relaxed. A nurse came to our room to offer us a morning break which, because the patient was stable, we did not refuse. My preceptor looked relieved to be able to sit down and enjoy a quick break, and I asked her if she had done many trauma cases. She replied that she had not, and she said "You just dive in and do what needs to be done for the patient." We returned to the room, finished the case and saw the patient safely to the intensive care unit. We then cleaned the OR room and prepared for the rest of the day's patients. I remember dwelling on what she had said to me. Here was a nurse that didn't do many trauma cases, yet you would have never known that from watching her. She remained calm and did whatever needed to be done to help save that patient's life that morning. I think about that day often. I think about watching the surgical team members bring order out of chaos, but, most of all I think about my preceptor, who was the best role model I could have had.

I knew within a year after nursing school that I eventually wanted to be an educator. With every new nurse for whom I was a preceptor, I would try to emulate the attitude of the preceptor I had when I was a student. And now that I am a perioperative staff educator, I keep that preceptor's words close to my heart. I remind all of our nurses that no matter what happens, keep your cool and do what's best for the patient.

Protecting Patient Confidentiality

Raphael J. "Ray" Landreneau, RN, BSN, CNOR
Baton Rouge, Louisiana

As a perioperative educator for the last 24 years, I am always looking for stories that convey the principles and concepts of our practice to use as teaching tools. The following story is one that I use in teaching new staff members how easily one can err and create an ugly confidentiality situation. It is a true story, but all persons' names have been changed for confidentiality.

A nurse named Mary was going to lunch at her hospital. She was an outstanding team member and had received several commendations for her more than 10 years of service at her institution. On her way to the cafeteria she passed the doors to the surgery department, and on this day, happened to see Jane, a woman from her church, being wheeled into the department. The nurse greeted her fellow church member, wished her well on her surgical outcome, and then Mary ended the short greeting by telling Jane she would be praying for her.

The next day Mary saw Helen, another member of her congregation. Mary mentioned to Helen to remember Jane in her prayers. She explained that Jane had had surgery the day before. Mary did not identify the type of surgery Jane was having, a fact Mary did not know. At this point one might think, "No harm, no foul," but that would be wrong.

Shortly after her conversation with Mary, Helen happened to encounter Jane's husband. He was alone at the time. As fate would have it, Helen asked about Jane and told him she had been praying for his wife. The husband looked at her quizzically. He had no idea what Helen was referring to. After a few questions, Jane's husband had some idea what had occurred. Jane had undergone a surgical procedure without her husband's knowledge. Jane became quite upset upon learning that this had been inadvertently revealed to her husband and demanded reparation from the hospital. Administrative personnel at the hospital decided that Mary's dismissal was warranted, and despite her previously impeccable record, they felt they had no choice but to appease the patient to avoid a lawsuit.

There are several important lessons to be learned from this incident. One, there was no malice or wrongful intent on the part of Mary. She meant no harm. In fact, her intentions were concern and caring for the patient. Unfortunately, her intent had nothing to do with the actual outcome or its effect on the patient. Even though Mary did not tell her friend Helen anything about the surgery, the fact that she revealed that Jane was receiving care at the hospital was enough to create a serious breach of confidentiality. Perioperative professionals must strictly adhere to the rules of confidentiality for all patients. The ultimate lesson is that you never know what may bring seemingly unrelated facts about a patient together in a disastrous way.

Providing Care Amidst Disaster

Louise Strickland RN, BN, CNOR
New York City, New York

I see the images on TV. It's not real to me yet. I know it is happening and people are hurting. But I am sitting in my comfortable apartment. After the earthquake hit Haiti, I found myself, like most, trying to find a way to help and feeling so useless at the same time. My boss called and said "I have something to ask you. Will you come to Haiti tomorrow?"

The next 24 hours passed in a blur. There was a flurry of activity to prepare anything and everything that would be needed, as little to no supplies would be provided in Haiti given the severity of the disaster. In past medical missions outside of the US that I have participated in, there was always a tie to the outside world, to a structure of stability. This was different—true devastation, true desperation. Concerns about what I would experience flashed through my mind as we approached the plane that would take us to a world torn apart.

When we arrived at the hospital in Haiti, near the city of Port-au-Prince, none of us were ready for what we saw. It was the worst situation I have ever seen. There were

13 of us in the group: two OR nurses, one trauma nurse practitioner, three orthopedic trauma surgeons, three trauma fellows, two anesthesia care providers, and two orthopedic implant consultants/scrub technologists.

The small community hospital in the hills overlooking Port-au-Prince was packed past capacity. The land around the hospital was covered with patients all lying on sheets, cardboard boxes, and pieces of wood. Some patients were just lying on the grass and dirt. Inside the hospital, it was no different. The hallways were crowded with around 750 patients and some family members. They all had injuries, mostly fractures, mostly open, and all infected. The smell of necrotic tissue was overpowering. The sight of these people and the suffering they had been through was overwhelming—it left nowhere for the mind to hide. We had to stay focused, however, and do everything we could for them. It had all become very real.

We brought our supplies with us and within about 30 minutes of arriving, we had two ORs up and running. The majority of the patients required amputations or external fixation of the fractures. Some needed debridement of their soft tissue wounds. With 40% of Haiti's population under 15, many of the patients we saw were children. Many of the patients were also pregnant women. This was particularly troubling, and we struggled to adjust to their great need.

In the four days we were there, we were able to perform around 120 surgeries, and we were able to save quite a few limbs because we had external fixation devices with us. We had to cut our time in Haiti short because a second plane full of supplies went missing between the airport and the hospital, and we were informed we would be given no further landing slots for supplies. One thing that touched all of us was the love and attention the families had for each other and their sick family members. They were so caring and sensitive to their needs, tending to them as best they could.

After returning home, the people of Haiti are still with me. I see them when I close my eyes. It's not easy to see people sick and suffering on such a large scale. To be able to care for those who have no other option for care really gave me a sense of being a true advocate for the patient. It gave me a sense of what is REALLY important and what is not. There are no prima donnas in these situations. There is no time or place for them.

Participating in a situation like this brought me back to the basics of OR nursing. I had to repeatedly ask myself, "What essentials do I need for this patient?" Sometimes it was a clamp or fresh scalpel, and sometimes it was offering a hand to hold or just a smile. It sounds clichéd, but an experience like this really puts things in perspective. Sometimes we can lose sight of the patient amongst all the paperwork, policies, and technology. This experience helped me be a better nurse when I returned to the US. I felt closer to my patients and to the core of why I first went into nursing 20 years ago.

Caring For a Pregnant Bariatric Patient

Rebecca Blades RN, BSN, CNOR, CRNFA
Kalamazoo, Michigan

As a perioperative nurse, I have the privilege and the responsibility to care for patients and provide them with a safe environment. Often, our work allows us to make a difference in someone's life. Recently, I was able to safely care for a pregnant mother and her unborn child, which was doubly rewarding.

I am the program leader for bariatric surgery at a community hospital. I am also a certified RN First Assistant (RNFA). On a recent morning, the medical director of the bariatric program told me that he had to cancel our morning meeting for the next day because he had added on a lap-band removal for a patient who was six months pregnant. I asked if he had consulted with the obstetric (OB) physician and the OB nursing staff about this patient's care. In addition to the mother's care, the fetus would need to be monitored preoperatively and postoperatively. I volunteered to look into arranging this for him.

In the process of making these arrangements, I discovered that this patient's OB physician did not have privileges at our hospital. When I told the surgeon this, he said he would just write the orders for the OB nurses to monitor the patient preoperatively and postoperatively. In doing so he would be responsible for interpreting the information the OB nurses collected. I asked him if he was comfortable with taking on this responsibility, and he was not. So, I recommended that he speak with our hospital's women's health services department personnel and ask them to consult during the patient's length of stay at our facility. This way we could be sure that both of the patients received the best care possible. He agreed and consulted our women's health services department. As a result, the patient and her baby were managed with the expertise of women's services as well as surgical services.

I then found the Society of American Gastrointestinal and Endoscopic Surgeons (SAGES) recommendations for care of the pregnant laparoscopic surgical patient and shared that information with the OR team. Used in conjunction with AORN's "Recommended practices for positioning the perioperative patient," we were able to position and care for the patient in the best and safest way for a pregnant patient. I also discovered that the CO_2 insufflation regulator on the laparoscopic machine should be set between 10 and 15 mm Hg and be kept at the lowest possible setting that provided a good visual field. Another bit of information I was able to share with the team is that, under the SAGES recommendations, tocolytic medications used for the treatment of preterm labor should not be used prophylactically for these patients.

I am so proud to have been a nurse patient advocate for both this patient and her fetus. I am sure that this patient will never know that nurses were looking out for her and her precious cargo, but it's all in a day's work for a perioperative nurse.

Sharing the Value of Aseptic Technique, Beyond the OR

Juanakee Pearson-Ceol, MS, RN
Columbus, Ohio

Today the perioperative field extends beyond the traditional OR. Hybrid suites are becoming common place and more invasive procedures are being performed by a broad group of health care professionals, such as interventional radiologists, with the assistance of radiology technologists.

As perioperative nurses, we sometimes take for granted that our knowledge and the way we focus on following recommended practices may not be the way that other health care professionals approach patient care. However, if we can find ways to share our knowledge in a way that is respectful and open, we can do a lot to promote perioperative nursing techniques that can be used to keep patients safe when receiving care outside of the OR. I learned this lesson first hand when I completed my master's degree and took a position as an educator in radiology. In entering this new area, I was eager to learn what I didn't know about the technology and the nonsurgical procedures patients were undergoing here.

Soon after beginning my work in radiology, I learned

that basic perioperative nursing skills, such as aseptic technique, were valuable to share with my new co-workers. In interventional radiology, technologists are not accustomed to using sterile technique to the magnitude we do in the OR. When I came to radiology I recognized that the environment was not what I was used to, particularly in areas designated as unrestricted, semi-restricted, and restricted. I also found that the approach to patient care in radiology was far more technical and linked to the procedure, rather than the more patient-centered approach perioperative nurses take.

When you come to a new work environment you pick and choose your battles. Nurses are still new to working in the radiology environment and serving as support staff members. As one of the few perioperative nurses in the area, I found myself in the minority. I knew that if I approached my new colleagues in radiology about aseptic technique and patient-centered care, I would have to do it in a way that wasn't judgmental or threatening. If I did not approach this correctly, I would end up alienating people and that would only be harmful to the patients.

Because the hospital where I work is a teaching institution, I decided that my best approach was to stick with evidence-based practice. Basic concepts of perioperative care such as aseptic technique are all based on evidence, and evidence transcends specialties. I prepared a program on "getting back to the basics of sterile technique." Sterile technique is vital to providing the patient with a safe environment, and it is relevant beyond the surgical setting. As part of this program, I shared information from AORN's "Recommended practices for aseptic technique," focusing on things like defining the principles of asepsis, opening a sterile package, and donning a sterile gown and gloves. I also focused on creating a sterile field and what to do if one's sterile field becomes contaminated.

By focusing my presentation on the evidence, and bringing AORN's recommended practices into our environment, I was able to provide my colleagues with knowledge that will help them improve the care they provide to patients, and that is something every health care professional wants to do. By presenting myself as open and wanting to provide evidence-based practices that could help all of us do our jobs better, I have been well received by my new radiology team. I not only provide a nursing perspective, I provide perioperative nursing resources to which they previously didn't have access. Today, if we have questions about safe care for the patient, I pull out my AORN *Perioperative Standards and Recommended Practices*, and we base our actions on these recommendations. The radiology team sees my presence as valuable because I am knowledgeable about procedures and the delivery of safe patient care. I am skilled to care for the whole patient, and I serve as a patient advocate. Caring for patients outside of the OR environment has unique challenges, but remembering to have an open mind and placing patient safety first are ways to promote the ideals of perioperative nursing, no matter what environment you are working in.

Understanding the Science Behind Sterile Processing

Rose Seavey, RN, BS, MBA, CNOR, ACSP
Denver, Colorado

S ometimes relations between the operating room and sterile processing can be like a bad marriage — there is a lack of communication and no one takes the time to really understand the issues and challenges the other faces. When the OR and the sterile processing department have bad relations, it is the patient who suffers. I have worked in both the OR and sterile processing. Doing this has given me a unique view into both worlds and has helped me to facilitate better collaboration between these partners.

For me, the key to understanding how these two departments can work together is to understand the science behind sterile processing. Surgical instruments are more complicated than ever before, with intricate parts and long narrow lumens. Because of the complexity of these devices, they sometimes require extended sterilization exposure time, as well as specific handling and packaging. It also is imperative that the manufacturer's written recommendations are followed to ensure sterility and patient safety.

Perioperative professionals may not understand the science behind safe sterility. The day this realization hit home for me was not long after I had made the jump from working in the OR to managing the sterile processing department in my facility. It was mid-morning when I got a call from a perioperative nurse requesting a bronchoscope. We had only sterilized the bronchoscope requested within the last hour, and I knew that any instrument sterilized with ethylene oxide (EtO) needs an aeration time of at least eight to 12 hours. I would have been remiss in my work if I had sent the instrument to the OR, and I had to explain this to the OR staff member requesting the instrument.

When I made the call to explain why the instrument could not be released yet, I thought about how many times I had called the sterile processing department from the OR asking, and often demanding, that they send an instrument I needed for surgery immediately. When I made these calls I was doing what I thought was best for my patient, and I was working on a tight OR schedule. I acknowledged these concerns when I explained to the OR staff member that the instrument needed more time to aerate the EtO. I explained the science behind this need for extended processing time. Ethylene oxide gas will remain on the product as well as the packaging unless it is appropriately aerated according to the manufacturer's recommendations. Ethylene oxide is a poisonous gas that may harm the patient or health care worker, if not completely aerated. The OR staff member understood my rationale for not sending the instrument after my explanation. Together we worked to come up with alternative instrumentation for the surgery that was sterile and ready for use. This incident marked the beginning of improved relations between the OR and sterile processing department personnel at my facility. We also began to include the OR staff members in our sterile processing in-services, and they did the same with us. By communicating our needs and by sharing our knowledge, we were able to begin operating as one large department, and this made all the difference for our patients.

Holding shared in-services leads to improved safety for our patients. Today, such collaboration is more important than ever, as The Joint Commission and the Centers for Medicare & Medicaid services take a stronger stand on the complete sterilization process in the OR.

As a consultant, I share sterile processing lessons I have learned with the OR staff and sterile processing staff members I talk to. Perioperative professionals and sterile processing specialists need to collaborate and share knowledge because it helps keep our patients safe—and that's something all of us can support.

Creating a 'Red Zone' in the OR

Sheila Haworth, RN
Savannah, Georgia

Despite the fact that loud noise and distraction should not be occurring in the operating room, perioperative nurses have all found themselves amongst chaos at the end of a surgical case when it's time to do a closing count. Loud music, ringing telephones, and casual conversation between staff members are distractions in the OR that can hinder accurate closing counts.

To combat this stressful atmosphere, our hospital has established a "Red Zone" in its ORs. The notion of a Red Zone started with the need to reduce medication errors in hospital units. It establishes a quiet, interruption-free zone around the automated medication dispensing machine we use, in which the nurse can focus on accurately preparing medications. It is known that distractions can cause mistakes. Medication errors are a serious safety issue in the medical profession. Our hospital did not take the problem lightly. The Red Zone has been an invaluable tool for many nursing units and can benefit other areas of the hospital as well.

In our hospital, it is the policy to extend the Red Zone

to the OR. At the beginning of the closing count, the Red Zone is established. The physician is then informed that the Red Zone has begun, radios are turned off, phones/pagers are left unanswered, and all unnecessary conversation ceases until the closing count has ended and is verified as correct. The circulating nurses and scrub technologists are responsible for maintaining the quiet environment while the count is being done.

I believe the suggestion for a Red Zone was well-received by management, who expedited a change in the closing count policy. There's also a feeling of empowerment among staff members because the Red Zone gives you the quiet time to get your thoughts together, get organized, and to help make an accurate closing count. The safety of the patient is our duty, and the Red Zone enables us to carry this out much more efficiently and with authority.

Fighting to Be a Nurse

Martha Baker, RN
Denver, Colorado

A t age 12, I asked an older friend of mine who was leaving for college what she planned to do there. She told me she was going to become a nurse. I asked her what that meant and when she told me, I decided I would follow in her footsteps and become a nurse, too. I went to high school and took the required courses. When my counselor asked where I would like to apply for college, I showed her a picture of Jersey City Medical Center, where I planned to study nursing. "You won't be able to go there," she said. When I asked why she replied, "Because they don't accept colored students." It was 1947, and this was not unusual.

I was determined to become a nurse. I graduated from high school and spoke to my mother about my plans for college. My mother said, "You won't be able to go to nursing school, we can't afford it." But I was determined. I got a job and saved enough money to pay my way through nursing school and, when the time came, I was accepted to the Jersey City Medical Center Nursing program.

I entered a class of 36 students that included five black

females—the first time this school had ever accepted this many black female students. My nursing education was not without unpleasant obstacles, but I persevered. I was so excited when it was time for me to do my OR clinical rotation. When I arrived in the OR, however, my new supervisor took me to the director of nurses and said, "She doesn't belong in the OR. She doesn't belong in nursing." By a stroke of luck, the OR supervisor's assistant decided to help me. She said, "Well let me spend a week with her and then we'll decide."

After my trial week in the OR was complete, the director's assistant took me back to the OR supervisor and said, "There's no reason why she can't complete the OR practical or her nursing education." The supervisor was not pleased, and I thought about quitting, but I had no money, no other occupation, and nursing was my passion. So I stuck it out and completed my practical in the OR, and my nursing education. I worked for one week at the hospital where I graduated. I found a job as a head nurse at the tuberculosis hospital connected to the Jersey City Medical Center complex. I was fortunate at this young age to be given a job as head nurse, but I was eager to get out and see the wider world.

Together with my nursing colleagues, we decided to enlist in the military. I applied to the Army and was accepted.

Three of us went on to active duty, but I'm the only one who stayed for 20 years. I retired in 1971 as a Lieutenant Colonel and a Vietnam veteran. When I retired from the Army, I wrote to the assistant OR supervisor who gave me a chance and gave me my first experience in the OR. I told her how grateful I was that she took the time to work with me. I told her that I did not know where I would be today if it wasn't for her kindness and her open mind.

I don't know if she ever received that note, but I still think about the path that led me to nursing. I think about the obstacles I overcame and the people who looked past the obstacles and saw the nurse that I could be. I think about how ironic it is that I spent such a wonderful career in the OR, a place so many people told me I didn't belong. My life has been full of ups and downs. I have fought adversity, prejudice, and other challenges along the way. But I thank God everyday that I fought to be a nurse—that I fought to work in the OR. In my profession I have met colleagues and patients along the way who have changed me, who have made me who I am. I am 82 years old. I continue to volunteer and enjoy life. I am so blessed.

Using a Checklist, Saving a Life

Elizabeth Norton, RN, BSN, CNOR
Boston, Massachusetts

I have been a staff nurse in the main operating room at a children's hospital for the past 24 years and additionally, I manage patient safety and quality for the OR. In 2004, I was appointed the hospital-wide champion for Universal Protocol as defined by The Joint Commission. This was an ideal role for me because I am passionate about patient safety and had already implemented "time out" and "site verification" in the main OR. When our institution adopted the World Health Organization (WHO) Surgical Safety Checklist in 2009 and modified it to meet the needs of a pediatric population, I was ready to facilitate the change.

My experience with using our checklist in the operating room has been both positive and rewarding. I have witnessed the checklist prevent potential errors and improve efficiency. The checklist prevents teams from relying on memory alone. By reviewing the checklist, the surgical team members are better prepared for surgery. For example, equipment needs during the surgery can be identified prior to the surgery. This has improved efficiency by giving the circulator the opportunity to obtain the items before they are needed.

By embedding "antibiotic prophylaxis" into our checklist, this automatically reminds the team to take this important safety step prior to incision, which helps prevent surgical site infections. Many times this has prompted staff members to review the time antibiotics were administered and to determine if another dose needed to be re-administered if the one hour pre-incision time frame had expired. This is an especially helpful reminder when a case has been delayed.

Human factors studies have shown that when team members use the names of surgical team members during critical events, it greatly improves patient outcomes. The simple addition of team introductions appears to have broken down social barriers and contributed to a better work environment. As surgical procedures become more complex, this checklist is proving to be very beneficial by fostering teamwork and communication. The checklist also prompts questions by team members and the traditional hierarchy (surgeon is the "captain of the ship") has been flattened.

I also have spoken with clinicians who resist the checklist. Some claim that they are already doing things that are included in the checklist, or that the introductions are not necessary because they already know the names of all team members. Others feel that the checklist takes too long and actually increases operative time. Additionally, there are clinicians who feel that bad things never happen to them. Many of these objections are often based in resistance to change; however, many clinicians also have witnessed the benefits of using the checklist and have adopted it into practice. Furthermore, each section of the checklist takes, on average, less than a minute to complete. The checklist is a low-budget, easy-to-complete initiative that improves efficiency and, in some cases, saves lives.

Checklists are not new to the perioperative environment. I implemented a preoperative safety checklist at our facility in 1999. We developed it to help prevent patients from entering the operating room unprepared, and it was a response to the newly implemented hospital requirement to mark the surgical site (this was prior to The Joint Commission requirement). We needed a checklist to help prevent patients from entering the OR until all preoperative surgical criteria were met and the surgical site was marked by the surgeon. The great thing about checklists is that they can be updated and modified to meet regulatory requirements or to incorporate changes that a facility feels are important.

Through auditing, we have seen that checklist compliance is high, and team members have expressed satisfaction with the flow and content of the checklist. Although our audits reflect strong compliance, we continue to strive to improve the quality of checklist use. For example, some team members may "skip" steps that they feel are non-applicable and some team members have committed the checklist to memory and don't use the printed version, which can lead to inadvertently missing some steps. We are working to improve compliance with the sign-out piece of the checklist, which lacks a clear trigger for teams to remember to complete it, and therefore it is sometimes left out of the workflow.

My advice to other colleagues striving to implement and refine surgical checklists is to obtain senior leadership support. Having support is crucial to implementing a surgical checklist. I have been asked by staff members at other hospitals how we manage resistance in performing this process. I usually reply by saying that involving leadership support for the checklist and having a well-established culture of patient safety helps everyone on staff accept the checklist as a standard of care. Collaborating with a multidisciplinary team also makes a big difference. I continue to work closely with both a surgeon and anesthesiologist who are highly committed to patient safety and to using the checklist. It also is important to involve front line staff members and routinely ask them for feedback about using the checklist. This constant feedback and ongoing dialogue makes staff members feel like they are part of the process and reduces resistance.

Education and follow up also are important elements of success. You can't simply roll out a checklist and expect it to work. You have to continue to educate team members, share data results, and find other solutions if proposed practices are not working. The more you talk about it, the more people realize it is workable and helpful to providing safe patient care.

As I look to the future, I can see that one surgical checklist may not fit every need. My vision for the future is that there will be an electronically generated, patient-specific surgical checklist tailored to meet the unique needs of each patient. For now, however, we must continue to refine the one-size-fits-all checklist that we have for the OR. Various types of checklists will continue to be developed and refined for ensuring safety and the complex care of patients in all aspects of medical care.

I will continue to promote the use of a checklist because

I am invested in providing quality care for each patient. Our work is complex and we are human, we can make mistakes, we can get distracted, and we can forget. A checklist is important if it can prevent adverse events or even save a life. I believe everyone wants to do a good job, and no one intentionally harms a patient. Our job is to advocate for the patient, and to keep them safe. Checklists can help us work as a team to give the best care possible.

Instilling Safe Medication Practices

C. Linda Wilkinson, RN, BSN, MA
Durham, North Carolina

"….What *IS* a 'milligram'?"

"I keep regular strength acetaminophen at home for my 12 year old. So I just double up and take 4 when I need pain relief for myself…"

"I can buy acetaminophen at the supermarket so it wouldn't be in my prescription medicine…would it?"

Understanding what our patients actually know about medication safety may challenge perioperative nurses to seriously consider what patients may not know about medication, but hesitate to ask in a health care setting. This can be especially relevant when planning patient education. As nurses, we are well aware that over-the-counter (OTC) preparations are "real" medicines, though patients may believe these are not important enough to mention. We now know that the potential for interaction among prescription medications and OTC drugs represents a significant health issue, but do patients? Over-the-counter products are available for purchase without the input or advice of a pharmacist or physician and may have serious consequences for patients. Medication safety is an important health issue and an opportunity, and a priority, for patient teaching.

Excessive use of acetaminophen in over-the-counter medicines and prescription drugs and its effects on the liver has been the subject of news headlines and was also discussed in the summer of 2009 at a US Food and Drug Administration (FDA) advisory committee meeting. In light of this, it is important to think about what we assume is common knowledge regarding acetaminophen, but which may not be understood by our patients. For example, we may know that APAP is the abbreviation for "acetaminophen," which appears on prescription-strength medication, but our patients may not know that. It is important to assess what a patient knows and how they take medication. For example, some patients may swallow a couple of extra-strength acetaminophen to give a 'boost' to their prescribed narcotic medication, and be unaware of the consequences.

This focus on medication safety is particularly important in an ambulatory surgical center (ASC) setting where patients are usually discharged far sooner than in the average inpatient setting. I have been a champion of the benefits associated with early postoperative discharge for myself, my children, and my patients. Positive patient outcomes for recovery, safety, comfort, and satisfaction are easily validated in ambulatory surgical centers. Yet ambulatory surgery significantly limits the time a nurse can spend on patient education following a surgical procedure.

We have been working with our patients to help them understand safe combinations of medicines that can be used to tackle postoperative pain and how to deal with and report pain that is not alleviated by prescribed medication.

We use a multimodal pain management plan and create individualized discharge care plans for all patients. These include information on widely used OTC medicines such as acetaminophen and ibuprofen, along with prescription medications such as nerve pain modulators and opioids. Medication safety thus presents extraordinary challenges to the knowledge, experience, and creativity of our nurses. It is our job to help patients make sense of medicines, whether these drugs are prescribed or found in their own medicine cabinets at home.

We inform patients that if their prescription medicine contains acetaminophen, they can *substitute* any OTC product also containing acetaminophen for the prescribed medication, but they should never *supplement* the medication with an OTC product. In our ASC, we are careful to tell patients exactly what is in their prescription, and we also try to determine what products they may use at home. We explain about the extra burden on the liver imposed by medicines, especially by acetaminophen, and educate patients about avoiding alcohol when using acetaminophen. We are careful to explain that products containing acetaminophen may contain between 325 mg and 650 mg per tablet. We then carefully review information about maximum total doses and how this translates into the numbers of pills it is safe to take.

We hope that the information we offer will prevent medication mishaps for our patients and that they will pass this information on to others. We believe that this patient education initiative enhances perioperative nursing practice with an opportunity for involvement in a timely public health issue.

Speaking Up for Safe Coordination of Patient Care

Grace Bascetta, RN, BSN, CNOR
Richmond, Virginia

I t's no secret that teamwork is the key to keeping our patients safe. Coordinating safe patient care among all members of the surgical team is not always easy, particularly when you are a new staff member trying to become accustomed to a facility's work flow, processes, and procedures. A good place to start laying the groundwork for open communication and teamwork is with perioperative nurses and surgical technologists.

Teamwork with fellow surgical team colleagues may seem a given, but this is often not the case. I learned this first hand when I took a position as RN circulator in a new facility. Unlike the work environment at my previous job, roles within the surgical team seemed more isolated in this new facility and some nurses tended to be territorial about their role and their approach to perioperative care. Early in my work at this new facility, I encountered a situation that led me to be more assertive in speaking up for my patient, both in my actions and in my communications with team members. This can be particularly hard when you are the new person at a facility.

I was the circulating nurse for a patient undergoing an inguinal hernia repair. In addition to me, there was a surgical technologist assigned to mentor a student technologist, a surgical assistant, the surgeon, and an anesthesia care provider. It was the start of the case, and I was counting with the student and waiting for the surgical technologist to scrub in. We had counted everything except the instruments. The surgeon arrived, and I told the student that I would count the instruments when the other technologist returned. The surgeon works fast and can be very impatient. He began asking for multiple items to get the case started. He wanted the implant, more sutures, and many other items. My time, the mentor's, and the student's were consumed getting the case started. In the middle of this activity, another nurse came in and said she was my lunch relief. I began explaining to her the patient information, where I was in the charting, and that I hadn't counted instruments. By this time, the doctor had inserted the implant and was closing.

As I continued to give the report, the other nurse said three times that I needed to go to lunch because she had three lunch reliefs to do. She said she would do what was needed to be done. I shouldn't have gone to lunch. When I came back from lunch the doctor was gone and the team was waiting for a radiologist to read the X-ray that had been taken to remedy the count irregularities: a drain was unaccounted for, and an extra suture package and a reel were present that were not on the count sheet. I felt I had been rushed to lunch, and my relief felt that she had been left with a disaster waiting to happen. She told me she was going to report me to the OR director and left.

After the X-ray revealed no retained drains, sponges,

instruments, suture needles or reels, and I transported the patient to the postanesthesia care unit with the anesthesia care provider, I wrote an incident report and stated that the instruments had not been counted before the operation.

I should have had all the instruments, sponges, needles, and instruments counted before bringing the patient into the OR. Because I didn't do that, I should have asked for help to get this done or to assist the surgeon to get the case started while I finished counting. I should not have put off counting the instruments. I should have insisted that the mentor was present from the start, and I should have told the relief nurse to come back and relieve me for lunch later so I could finish my responsibilities first. I should have taken my patient's best interests into consideration first and not allowed myself to be forced to leave for lunch when I was not prepared to do so. I did not use good judgment when I decided to put off counting the instruments. I should have insisted that the student surgical technologist's mentor be present during set up and counting and I should have finished the count before leaving for lunch. Later in the day the director called me into her office. She was very understanding. Together we discussed what occurred and how I could approach a situation like this in the future. This incident also reminded me how important it is to speak up and to do what I know is right.

Nurses need to communicate incidents to their managers. If they need help, they can't wait until a situation gets worse and the patient's safety is compromised. New nurses should feel comfortable calling for assistance and they should stand up for themselves, even when the situation is uncomfortable because their patient's safety is at stake.

Acknowledging the Triumphs and the Challenges our Colleagues Face

Maureen Melia Chadwick, RN, MSN, NE-BC
Erie, Pennsylvania

Each of us comes to work fighting some personal battle—maybe it's a personal challenge such as caring for parents, keeping our children on task in life, or trying to support our loved ones. Distractions and stressors in our personal lives can sometimes spill over into our professional lives and potentially compromise patient safety. As a perioperative director, I consider it part of my role to be coach, confidant, and listener, because serving staff members in this way can help them to better focus their attention on the patients and procedures. It is more important than ever that we are laser-focused on the task at hand in the operating suite.

This approach has helped me to listen more and to pick up on the nuances that may trigger further conversation to uncover the stressors that staff members are up against. One experience in particular with a fellow nurse* has made me think twice when talking with staff members and has led me to ask myself, "What personal battle is this individual fighting that I may not even be aware of?"

This nurse's personal battle is breast cancer. On a very

personal level, her battle is one I may face some day, as my mother and aunt are breast cancer survivors, and their youngest sister died of cancer at 48. Despite this battle, I have witnessed the attention this nurse gives to her work, the patients who come through the OR suites, her many co-workers, and her family. Additionally, watching her in her new role as a patient has provided insight to me as a leader in health care. She is the specialty resource nurse for neurosurgery at our hospital. Not only was she instrumental in defining the role of specialty resource nurse for all specialties, but she is a role model for all nurses in this position. She is an incredible person, a great mother and nurse, and a good friend. Her clinical practice is just one of the many examples of her excellence, and she sets the bar very high for nursing practice in the operating room.

A specialty resource nurse leads the specialty team he or she is responsible for, and in this instance it is the neurosurgical team. She is first and foremost the patients' advocate by assuring patient safety in all aspects of care and reassuring those patients who may feel anxious prior to surgery. In the OR she assures proper positioning of patients, she checks the instrument trays for each of her patients, and she conducts what we call the "final time out" before surgery. She leads the call for everyone in the OR to check their role and focus on the surgery at hand.

Her nursing approach is "no nonsense" for all members of the perioperative team. Anytime we implement a new practice or procedure, the surgeons look to this nurse for her approval. She assures them that they have everything they need for each and every surgical procedure. And while she can be one tough cookie, she also has a great sense of humor and even on the most challenging days can find something to laugh about to lighten the mood.

January 16, 2009, became one of the most challenging days in her life. She was diagnosed with breast cancer at 38 years of age. I still remember the day she was waiting to hear the diagnosis. I knew the minute she walked into my office what the diagnosis was without her saying the word "cancer." She shed a few tears at that moment—in fact, we both did. Minutes later, however, her positive approach to life emerged as she was determined to fight back.

She underwent her first surgery thirteen days later and returned to work in less than two weeks. Another surgery was scheduled two weeks after that, and she again returned to work after a short recovery period. When radiation treatments began, her primary care nurse asked if she planned to work through her treatments. There were 33 treatments planned, and she worked full time, went to the gym three to four times a week, and attended all the softball and soccer games for her two teenage girls. Toward the end of these treatments it was clear they were taking their toll, and while she never complained, I knew how exhausted she was. She continued to persevere through, which was an inspiration to everyone who knew her.

I didn't know this nurse until I became the director in the operating room, and it is interesting how our lives cross paths with others'. After getting to know each other, we found out we both live in the same part of town, like to hang out at the same places, and have been through some of the same experiences in life.

While 2010 was to be a fresh start for this nurse, it was almost a year to the day that a follow-up mammogram revealed another calcification, which upon biopsy turned out to be precancerous cells. She underwent surgery on

January 28, 2010, and while the surgery seemed to progress smoothly, upon waking up she learned that the needle localization done prior to surgery that morning had slipped away from the biopsy site, and the surgeon was not certain she had taken a biopsy from the correct site. That meant the nurse needed to come back for more surgery. I was able to be with her in the postanesthesia care unit, and her tears echoed the frustration we all felt. She is not one to shed tears easily. I knew she was ready to move on from this chapter in her life, but that was not to be. What I have learned is that, while we take many steps to assure that procedures go well, mistakes still can happen. To watch this happen to a friend is difficult. This has reinforced to me that for the average patient who doesn't understand health care, it is important to take extra time to explain why something like this has happened.

I am happy to report that my friend is now cancer free. She takes nothing for granted and I continue to support her. It is truly an honor to work with her. She is a role model for nursing, but also for any woman facing this disease. I also appreciate the other nurses, physicians, and perioperative staff members I work with who may be experiencing personal struggles in silence. I encourage all staff members to find support for themselves and their patients. I also encourage perioperative leaders to step back and acknowledge the human side of their staff members—to realize that everyone we work with is facing his or her own battles. Recognizing each others' personal and professional struggles and successes helps all of us provide better care for our patients.

*Permission was granted by the nurse discussed in this story.

Recognizing the Human Factor

Charlotte Guglielmi, RN, BSN, MA, CNOR
Boston, Massachusetts

We often view leadership as something we do with our head, but experienced leaders know that leadership must also come from the heart. As leaders, we put into place the tools that staff members need to make a difference for patients. We develop guidelines and policies to guide staff members in making decisions. It's easy for leaders to see policies and procedures as stop gaps that mitigate error. Relying on these stop gaps is an example of leading only with the head because we know that stop gaps don't always address the human factor.

I was reminded of this when my facility had a wrong site surgery. We thought we had fail-safe policies in place and years of audit data led us to believe we were protected against error. This false sense of security led to an event that not only harmed a patient, but also affected all those caring for the patient.

When any error occurs in a health care setting, there are multiple victims. The patient is obviously our biggest concern. As a leader, it is important to recognize that staff members and even the institution are also victims, because an error opens staff members and the facility to scrutiny, and it makes everyone question the system and its ability to provide safe care. In the end, this is a good thing, but the process is difficult. It's heart wrenching when you believe you have everything in place for safe care, only to have to find where things went wrong.

I can recall the day this wrong site surgery occurred like it was yesterday. It was at the end of June during the annual change-over of medical house staff. Those of us who work in academic centers know this is a time of chaos as new fellows, residents and interns rotate between several facilities within our hospital system. This process can be especially confusing because each facility has its own set of policies and procedures, creating a situation where standard practice in one facility may be different from standard practice in another.

I was in a planning meeting with perioperative leadership, the surgical chief of quality, and the clinical director of anesthesia when all of our beepers went off. The text message read that a wrong site surgery had just occurred. We were shocked. It was everyone's worst nightmare—having a patient wake up and ask, "why do I have a cast on this foot?" The first thing we did was head to the site of the error to check on the patient and to support the surgeon during the initial disclosure discussion. Then we turned to supporting the staff members and physicians involved with this wrong site surgery. The event was discovered around noon; by 4 p.m. we had assembled the entire team, including the Chief of Nursing, surgical chiefs of staff, health care quality leadership, perioperative leadership personnel, and members of the surgical team.

We also included social workers with expertise in crisis management. Together, we debriefed every step of the patient's care.

This process was difficult. I had to look at the situation with my heart and my head. From a logical perspective, I had to understand each step of the patient's care to find what went wrong. I had to approach my colleagues with compassion, while asking them tough questions and expecting honest answers. I had to understand staff dynamics to know how they would react in a crisis and if any staff members had a history of disregarding policy. As we all discussed this event, we could see, in hindsight, how one event led to another. While the team was focused on the technical aspects of this procedure that is only done a few times a year in our facility, we learned that staff members did not perform the time out, although they thought they did. We also learned that the music playing in the OR distracted staff members. We saw where these factors and other failures occurred that led to this wrong site surgery.

Thankfully, good things have come from this event. First and foremost, we took immediate care of the patient which included full disclosure and support. Also, this event and the debriefing process that followed brought the surgical team closer together because they had to look critically at their own role in this event and also how their role was integrated with the actions of other team members. This event and debriefing experience led to the creation of a safety culture task force responsible for reviewing policies and procedures to ensure they make sense to every staff member in the OR. Task force members also have worked to create greater standardization for the facility's preoperative safety processes, including changes to the way the team conducts the time out. For example, we put a structured, role-specific scripted time out in place to enable all members of the surgical team to articulate necessary information and also to feel comfortable participating in open dialogue as part of this safety check.

Members of this safety culture task force also said they did not want the radios on in the OR during the final time out because they wanted to be able to ensure they can hear all communication among members of the team. They also take the opportunity to review wrong site surgeries that occur at other facilities as a way to learn from the error and to look at how this could happen at our facility. I am proud of my colleagues for having the courage to recognize failure and learn from it in a way that has improved safety practices. In doing this, all of us had to recognize the needs of our hearts and our heads. As one of their leaders, it was my job to listen to them and guide them in this process.

I believe every perioperative nurse is a leader. I also believe we must look for the good in difficult situations. Every day we work for our patients, we work to keep them safe and this takes both knowledge and compassion. In my work as a perioperative leader, I lead with my head, but I also allow my heart to engage in the humanness of the incredible work we do.

Remembering to Believe

Jane Klein, RN
Denver, Colorado

Working in the OR, I have witnessed some very tragic injuries and their outcomes. I find myself wondering why bad things happen to good people and I find myself questioning why painful things happen to us in this life. During the last year I have lost two very important people. I do not understand why these things happen, but I truly believe that God takes care of fragile hearts and eventually helps us to accept the pain of our loss. In addition to the tragedies I have seen, I also have witnessed miracles in the OR that I remember when I am faced with events that are difficult to understand.

One Saturday morning we were performing surgery on a young man from Nebraska who had been stabbed in the heart. He was originally diagnosed with superficial wounds and as his condition worsened, he was flown to our hospital for treatment. The emergency response team transported him directly to the OR from the helipad and the surgeon opened his chest to discover that the stab wound had occurred where his aorta ascended out of his heart. In trying

to repair this fragile area, it became obvious that the patient
would need heart bypass to allow the surgeon to repair
the injury. We called a nearby university medical center
and tried to arrange for the patient's transfer; however, the
bypass team was in the midst of a bypass case and had
another one to follow and could not accept the patient. In
an attempt to save his life, one of the cardiac surgeons from
the university came to our facility to help. While we were
waiting for him to arrive, the patient's chest was packed and
closed to slow the bleeding by tamponade. Our attending
surgeon left the room to tell the patient's parents that
their son's injury was very grave and that he probably had
sustained a life-ending injury. Their only request was that
he be baptized while in the OR and still living.

In the interim, the cardiac surgeon from the university
had arrived and scrubbed in. The surgeons re-opened the
patient's chest and attempted to suture the area of the
heart and aorta involved. Unfortunately, this caused more
bleeding and tearing to the tissue. The patient's pressure
had dropped to 40 mmHg, his hematocrit was very low, and
his heart rate was about 140 beats per minute. The priest
we had summoned came into the room very quietly, and I
gave him some water with which to anoint the patient. He
stepped to the head of the bed, and baptized the patient.
The surgeon announced all of a sudden that the bleeding
had stopped. The patient's pressure began to improve and
his heart rate started to slow. The surgical team was able
to close his chest, and we safely transported him to the
intensive care unit. Surprisingly, the patient ended up going
home with his family in about one week.

I later shared with the attending surgeon the timing of
the baptism. The surgeon was not aware of the baptism or

the presence of the priest, but the expression on her face said it all. I believe that the patient was blessed, and that miracles do happen.

I share this story for those who question their faith and the ways of the world within the OR and beyond. I remember this patient, who was at the brink of death and is now with his family, and my faith is renewed. It has helped me do the best job I can, knowing that as long as I do my best the rest is out of my control. I believe that God provides for us in his own way, in his own time. My faith helps me in the OR. It helps me to believe in what we do to keep our patients safe, and to remember what is beyond our control.

Interpreting Care for Patient and Family

Kristy P. Simmons, RN, CNOR
Baton Rouge, Louisiana

It was a routine Monday morning in the Neonatal Intensive Care Unit Operating Room (NICU OR) when we received a call that we would have another emergency case added on. Prior to checking this new patient into the OR, I learned that the mother of the infant needing surgery only spoke a foreign language. She had just been discharged from the hospital herself and she was trying to locate the father of the child who could speak English, but had not been able to get in touch with him yet. I told the unit secretary that I would need our facility's Language Line interpretation service set up for my preoperative interview just in case the father was not here prior to the start of surgery.

The surgical patient was a two-day-old Hispanic infant presenting with vomiting induced by feeding. The diagnosis was pyloric stenosis. This defect required emergency laparoscopic pyloromyotomy surgery to correct the defect. Prior to surgery, the infant was accompanied to the surgical unit by his mother only because the patient's father was out in the field on a job and could not be located.

As I began to interview the mother of the infant, she informed me "no English" so we accessed our Language Line to help with the language barrier. The Language Line helped me connect with an interpreter for my preoperative interview so the patient's mom and I could discuss her infant's medical history, and I could verify that the mother understood the urgency of the situation and the need for immediate surgery.

The surgeon was in a hurry, and he came in the room asking what the hold-up was, trying to rush my surgical interview. He stated he had already spoken to the mom and was ready for surgery to start NOW! I told him it was going to take me a couple of more minutes—refusing to be rushed in my preoperative interview. I told him that, as the circulating nurse, it is my responsibility to verify identity of the patient, obtain patient and family medical history, inform the parents of pediatric patients of the procedure that will be performed, verify surgical consents, identify the surgical site and answer any questions the parents may have, using the AORN guidelines.

Of course it took us a few minutes to get the Language Line set up, and it was hard to ignore the surgeon and avoid rushing through the preoperative process when he was behind me tapping his toe, trying to speed up the preoperative interview.

However, I persevered with the interview. As I began my questioning with the infant's mother through the Language Line, her facial expressions became more and more stressed with each question I asked, and she started visibly shaking and hugging her infant more tightly toward her chest. As a mother myself, I understood her emotions and had nothing but empathy for her facing an emergency medical situation for her newborn infant, and not able to understand a word of the language being spoken all around her. I also understood a few extra seconds now could change her whole outlook on this hospital experience and on the nurses that work in the operating room.

As a nurse and a mother of four children myself, I could only imagine what I would be feeling if I were faced with the same situation. With another query from the surgeon on what was taking so long, I informed him I was going to be a few more minutes because I needed to reassure the mother that her child was going to be taken care of, and I was going to treat this patient as all of my other patients and complete a thorough preoperative interview. Just because the mother could not speak English was no excuse for me to rush back to the OR.

When I returned back to the Language Line with the mother of the infant, it looked like she was terrified and about to fall apart. I did not know how much of our conversation she had understood so I told the interpreter to tell the mother of the infant that I would treat her infant as though he was my own baby, until I could place him safely back into her hands. I also told the interpreter I was going to put the phone down for a minute because I felt like the mother needed a hug. As these words were relayed to her by the interpreter, I could see her shoulders relax and the tension disappear. As I hugged her she started to cry and repeated one of the few words I understood in her language over and over again, which meant: "Thank you, thank you."

This was an uncertain situation for both the infant and the mother, but as a nurse I had the obligation to be the patient advocate and take my time with the mother of the infant to reduce her anxiety and fears. I also needed to explain to the surgeon that I needed a few more minutes with my patient and his mother prior to the surgical intervention. I had informed the surgeon it would be a couple of extra minutes to interview the patient through the Language Line, but that it was important for the mother of the child to understand what I was saying and to have the same standard of care that I provide to all other surgical patients.

Sometimes the best thing to do in an emergency situation is to treat patients as you and your family would want to be treated in the same situation. I only wish I had a picture of the smile on the mom's face when I returned her child to her after surgery.

Learning from Loss

Barbara L. DiTullio, RN, BSN, MA
Boston, Massachusetts

It was late afternoon in June of 2005, and the surgery began just as countless other previous total knee replacement procedures had. The surgical team expected the patient, not yet 50 years old, to undergo the procedure without problems and wake up with improved knee function. Despite his complex past medical history, we had no reason to expect he would not survive the surgery, yet he did not. The team worked diligently for nearly two hours to prevent his death and none of the clinicians present were prepared for it. We were devastated. The surgeon, deeply affected by the outcome, cancelled the remainder of his surgical schedule.

For most members of the team, this was their first experience with a death in the OR. The group was upset and tearful. Many recalled family members who had passed—a normal reaction to the situation. There were many new practitioners present during the surgery, including newly-licensed nurses and technologists. The nurse manager on duty, a seasoned member of the staff, helped prepare the patient for the morgue. The team handled the situation well and left at the end of the day exhausted, but okay given the experience they had endured.

The following morning, the group was serious, but able to share their feelings quite openly. One new nurse said she was fine but couldn't stop crying. Another couldn't get the face of a person on whom he had initiated CPR in a public place out of his mind. This loss represented a new beginning because this group became the first to benefit from a pilot study providing peer support to help staff members deal with their emotions after an upsetting event. The intent was to provide caregivers an opportunity to come together as a team and debrief in a safe forum where they could discuss their feelings. Staff members were initially reluctant to do this, expressing fear of personal and professional safety, but all were assured this was solely for their benefit and strictly confidential. The group met privately for nearly two hours and, in the midst of their tears, they had time and space to reflect. In doing so they supported each other. The caregivers still needed time to process and heal, but each left with a lightened load that day.

Nearly five years have passed since the events of that day, yet they remain fresh in my mind. The loss of this patient, the debriefing, and countless other losses have profoundly changed me as a manager and influenced the way I view my role. I have learned many important lessons along the way.

I have learned that every caregiver has a professional face—a persona that performs as expected in a given clinical situation. However, underneath the professional face and frequently stoic veneer is a person who is susceptible to hurt from their experiences. We show up each day, work hard to make a difference in the lives of our patients, and in the end we must be prepared for the emotions that come with the level of care and dedication we provide. We also want to be valued for what we bring to the table.

I have learned to appreciate the privilege that my present work affords me—the opportunity to work with patients through critical times in their lives and the opportunity to work with staff members to participate in debriefings about clinical, interpersonal, and other work-related concerns. In every situation, something extraordinary happens when you assemble a group of individuals around a table and provide space and time to allow people to speak their truth. Despite the awkward apprehensions about the debriefing process we established that day, we found that people find a way to reflect and discard assumptions, misperceptions, and misunderstandings to get to a place that is invariably much better and brighter.

It is said that nothing comes into our experience without our invitation. Although not everyone embraces this idea, every experience comes with a lesson. For better or worse, the lessons teach. My fellow perioperative nurse, Patricia Seifert, says, with such wisdom and grace, that she has come to believe the worst of situations, and the best of people. I find myself a humble student of this philosophy.

Holding your Ground

Julie A. Martin, RN, BSN, MBA
Denver, Colorado

Most of my 23 years in nursing have been in the perioperative arena in a leadership role. Being an advocate for patient safety is not always easy, especially as it relates to difficult surgeons and a lack of effective communication in the OR. While this story is not about a patient specifically, the courageous conversation that occurred affected communication between nurses and a surgeon in the OR and increased staff confidence. This in turn has helped ensure patient safety going forward.

Everyone has unpleasant colleagues they must try to work with. Sometimes this person is a surgeon who may be mean and nasty and who everyone hates to work with. That was the case early in my career when I worked on a heart team in a major metropolitan area. Several of the surgeons on this team were wonderful to work with—collegial, respectful, and enjoyable. Working with one surgeon, however, was extremely difficult. Being assigned to work in a room with him immediately raised my anxiety level. I was afraid to ask any questions during the surgery. In fact

"Doctor Heartless," as he was covertly nicknamed, was so unbearable that team members kept a roster to ensure that no one had to work with him on a regular basis.

One day I was working as the charge nurse, and one of the perfusionists informed me that a patient was "crumping" in the cardiac catheterization laboratory. I called Doctor Heartless to verify if we should open the OR room and prepare for surgery. I cannot repeat the profanity and yelling that ensued over the phone; but more worrisome to me, he informed me that he was on his way down "to deal with me!" My instincts told me to run, but the professional nurse in me was up for the challenge. I was tired of dealing with his unprofessional behavior, as was the team.

The surgeon seemed to fly down the hall toward me, yelling at me as he approached, his face turning an unhealthy shade of purplish red. I said nothing while he ranted and when he finally stopped, I informed him that when he calmed down and could have a professional conversation with me I would be waiting for him. I really thought he might hit me! Another round of verbal abuse spewed out of his mouth before he stomped off. Fortunately, the patient did not have to come to the OR, and I saw no more of the surgeon that day. I informed the OR director the next day that I would not tolerate his behavior any more. The director stood up for me and told the surgeon he had to apologize to me. This happened a week later when he finally calmed down.

I still remember meeting with that surgeon in my office. When he began to verbally abuse me again I managed to get a few words in. I asked him, "Do you know that your entire team hates working with you and that we keep a list and rotate team members who have to work with you?! You are so unapproachable that we are afraid to ask you any questions and that is affecting the care of your patients!" For some unknown reason he stopped dead in his tracks, became very silent, and looked so defeated. He said, "I had no idea," and he walked away.

The next day, he found me again and we had the first real conversation in my two years of working with him. He apologized to me, saying "I had no idea that is what my team thinks of me." I replied, "Please don't just apologize to me, apologize to the team. They have had to tolerate this behavior far longer than I have." Not only did he apologize but his behavior changed significantly.

That was a defining moment in my perioperative leadership career. Maybe it's because I have a sister who was a physician and I considered her a colleague and not my superior, but I have never allowed a physician to bully or demonstrate inappropriate behavior in the operating rooms I supervise. I encourage even novice nurses to always give and expect respect from all team members, regardless of their roles. There are too many things that can go awry when caring for patients in such a stressful environment, and there is no room for ineffective or abusive communication. Thank goodness younger physicians are exposed to communication and team training education and are much less likely to behave abusively.

You may not always be rewarded immediately for standing up to this type of behavior and trying to stop it. Sometimes, however, your actions can significantly change a relationship for the better. The surgeon in question suffered a stroke several months later and came to me in the OR to ask for help because he felt "something was wrong."

He had come to respect me for the nursing skills I possessed and felt that he could come to me for help. It was very humbling. I accompanied him to radiology and stayed with him while he needed me. We are all human, even surgeons. Some of us just need occasional reminders.

Thinking Critically, for All Cases

Jane Buysse Fox, RN, CNOR
Minneapolis, Minnesota

While this event happened 20 years ago, it seems like yesterday when I talk about it. As I think about my experiences with this patient, I still get tears in my eyes.

I had a great assignment for the afternoon: OR 1, mediastinoscopy—a straightforward case I was comfortable circulating for. We pulled the case cart into the OR, and I went off to the preoperative area to visit and interview my patient, a young woman in her 30's named Katie (fictitious name). I introduced myself and instantly felt a strong connection with the patient. I felt like I had known her and her husband for years and was reconnecting with them rather than meeting them for the first time. They appeared so in love and happy with life as they easily shared stories with me about their two young daughters and their dogs.

Once Katie was transported to the operating room I introduced her to the scrub person, and we chatted until the anesthesia care provider was ready for induction. I was at her side as she drifted off to sleep—peacefully entrusting us with her care. The surgical team draped her and began her surgery. Within minutes, we were in crisis mode when the scrub nurse suddenly yelled, "Jane, the suction, we're bleeding!" I looked up from my charting to see the suction canister filling up as if it was under an open faucet. I called for help. The anesthesia care provider paged any available cardiac surgeon STAT to OR 1. In the blink of an eye another anesthesia care provider, as well as a cardiovascular surgeon, arrived to help, accompanied by an entourage of other staff members. This case had turned from routine to life-threatening in seconds.

An additional cardiac surgeon scrubbed in and the patient's chest was opened. I could see that the cell saver suction was filling quickly. Finally, after what seemed like an eternity, the surgeon located the bleeding site. A large tumor had displaced the innominate artery and was the primary bleeding site. Eventually the surgeon got the bleeding under control, but not until the anesthesia care provider had infused several units of blood to save this young woman's life. What I had just experienced was team work in the OR at its finest.

I felt a responsibility to stay near Katie to help with her care, as this event had happened under my watch. The charge nurse, who had kept in touch throughout our situation, asked me several times, "Are you OK? You are white as a sheet." "No," I said. "I'm fine." Only later when I looked at myself in the mirror did I see a pair of blue eyes staring back at me from a face void of any color. When I was relieved at the end of my shift it was difficult to pry myself from the operating room to go home.

Later that evening, I called in to find out what had happened to Katie. I learned she was out of the OR, and the team had transferred her directly to the postoperative cardiac care unit. I returned to work at 6:30 a.m. the following day and quickly changed into scrubs. As soon as possible, I went to check on Katie. Her husband sat in the chair next to her bedside, and they both greeted me. Her husband said "Good morning, how are you today? I understand she gave you quite a scare yesterday."

What an understatement, I thought. As I placed my hand on his shoulder I replied with tears in my eyes, "You are so lucky to have her here with you today." He smiled and said, "I should have told you this family likes drama; her father was scheduled for open heart surgery a few years ago and as we arrived to see him before surgery, he coded! He was taken immediately to surgery." Luckily the father recovered well from his open heart surgery. We chatted for a few minutes, and I returned to the OR. I continued to make daily visits and wished her well with her recovery. Sadly, the diagnosis had been grim, so I knew that she would be back for further care. I kept track of her thereafter until her death from the metastatic lung tumor about a year later.

Katie's mediastinoscopy procedure took place in the fall of that year, and at Christmas we received a beautiful red poinsettia with a card addressed to the OR. It read, "Thanks for taking such good care of our Mommy!" and was signed by Katie's daughters. It brought tears to my eyes and to the staff members involved in her case. She was a mother, a wife, and she was appreciative of everything we did for her.

I relate this story to all new nurses in the OR because it is a prime example that all cases in the OR can change rapidly, creating the need for critical thinking skills and quick actions to turn a life-threatening situation around, and that it takes a team to accomplish it.

Advocating Health Awareness Abroad

Valerie Kirchmann, BS, RN, CNOR
and Sandy Lapin, RN
New York City, New York

Like many people, we have both been affected by breast cancer. As nurses, we felt a strong need to educate about awareness and early detection of this disease, here at home and abroad. Our journey for this mission began in 2008 when we decided to do a poster presentation on breast cancer awareness in the lobby of our hospital as part of Perioperative Nurse Week. During this poster presentation, we realized the need to educate women and men about breast cancer awareness within the hospital, and also in the community.

As fate would have it, a surgical resident at our hospital had a dream about taking breast cancer awareness to Ecuador, where breast cancer is on the rise. This doctor spoke to the OR staff about her project and the need for volunteers. We immediately volunteered and went to work writing fundraising letters to get donations from corporations and health care professionals. Volunteers for this educational mission included medical students, residents, a physician's assistant, and others who made up our multidisciplinary effort with each person contributing his or her unique skills.

We held meetings and made plans. As with any project there were problems, but when you have a dream and determination nothing can stop you. Soon a group of dedicated volunteers left for Ecuador, our luggage packed to the brim with donations. Some of the group left earlier to set the groundwork for the team. We arrived in Santiago de Guayaquil, a large city in Ecuador, and were briefly detained due to customs issues. We were allowed to travel in Ecuador after obtaining help from the American Consulate. A short flight brought us to the city of Cuenca where we spent the night. Our team finally reached our destination of Gualaceo—a village of 40,000 people located in the Andes the following day. Gualaceo is a pretty village with a beautiful church in the center and an open-air market.

After getting settled in a nearby hostel, the team set up a registry at the church where local patients received breast and general health examinations in cubicles surrounded by shower curtains for privacy. We referred some patients to the local hospital in Gualaceo, where treatment areas were set up for biopsies and surgery. A few of the women would do their handcrafts while waiting to be seen. Their crafts included sweaters and scarves knit with fine wool and were colorful and exquisitely done.

The team members served more than 1,000 women and men from nearby areas by the end of the week. More and more villagers came each day, and by the last day, we had to call in the military for crowd control. We taught patients about breast self exams and breast care, including visual instructions about how to palpate and "find the lumps," and we gave out posters and brochures for them to keep. One patient took the information to her village to teach the women there about breast care. She had walked hours to reach us at the Gualaceo hospital and get the information to share with her community.

The Gualaceo hospital has very limited resources, but all staff members were dedicated to their patients. They worked with what they had available. One night while we were assisting during a lumpectomy, the lights and water went out. We learned this is a regular occurrence at the hospital. A flood light and a suction machine shared between anesthesia and the surgeon enabled the team to complete the surgery. Next door, volunteers from our group also delivered a child in the dark.

Each night we returned to the hostel tired but with a sense of accomplishment, knowing that we helped people and taught them to take control of their health. Early breast cancer detection saves lives and that was the continuing message we promoted. On our last day there, we all agreed this trip would be just the start of an ongoing relationship with the Gualaceo Hospital.

Before we left for Ecuador people asked, "Why leave the United States when we have breast cancer education needs here at home?" Our answer was "Why not?" Breast cancer is a global concern. No one is immune and early detection does save lives. Fighting a disease like breast cancer requires a global effort to educate and seek a cure. Rainforests such as those in Ecuador may hold the answer for finding a cure. Perhaps one of the women we helped will have a child—perhaps the baby born that night in the dark—who will discover a cure for breast cancer. Hope is universal, and we must have it and believe in it for a better world. The experience was incredibly empowering. It allowed us to provide the men and women of the Gualaceo community and beyond with the knowledge to protect themselves and to provide them with the tools to educate their community about health and breast cancer awareness.

Remaining Focused Through a Trauma Case

Stella Harrington, RN, BSN, CNOR
Boston, Massachusetts

I work at a Level 1 Trauma Center, so I am accustomed to providing emergency care to pediatric patients who have sustained a serious or critical bodily injury as a result of a fall or car accident. However, nothing could have prepared me for an 11-year-old girl who arrived in the OR one Sunday morning in September with violent trauma injuries.

Around 6:30 a.m. the nurses working the night shift received a STAT page stating that an 11-year-old girl with stab wounds was en route to our facility—estimated time of arrival: 20 minutes. The nurses, unsure as to where the stab wounds were located or the severity of the wounds, spoke with the attending anesthesiologist about setting up an operating room. They then gathered the supplies and equipment needed for the procedure. We put all the cases scheduled for the assigned trauma room on hold until it was decided whether the patient would be coming to the OR. The anesthesia fellow went down to the ER to ascertain if the patient had arrived.

At approximately 8:00 a.m. the anesthesia fellow

returned to the OR and informed us that the patient had
arrived and had sustained multiple stab wounds all over
her body. Not knowing which part of her body we would
be operating on or which surgical service/surgeons would
be operating on the patient, we assembled supplies and
equipment in anticipation of a major abdominal surgery,
as well as a general/chest/cardiac case with plastic and
orthopedic surgery likely needed, as well.

At approximately 8:30 a.m., we knew the patient was
in the ER but did not know if she would be coming to the
OR. My first thought was that the stab wounds must not be
too severe or she would have been brought to the OR right
away. The other two nurses and I discussed the need to
proceed with the other surgical cases scheduled for the day.
I discovered that the patient was in CAT scan and called for
information. I was informed that the patient had left and
was now in X-ray. X-ray personnel informed me that the
patient had left and had returned to the ER. I relayed all of
this information to the charge nurse. She called the ER and
asked to speak to the ER charge nurse who informed her
that the patient was stable and had been placed in a Level 9
Category. A level 9 situation means that information cannot
be shared with anyone calling from outside the hospital.
Anyone calling for information is to be told that we did not
have any information regarding the patient.

The ER charge nurse also explained that the patient's
mother had been killed during the home invasion, during
which the patient had been stabbed and that the patient did
not know that her mother had died. Part of the discussion
in the ER centered on locating the father, who was away on
a business trip, to obtain surgical and anesthesia consents.
In the end, the decision was made to send the patient to the

OR. It was decided that I would circulate and the other two nurses would scrub.

The patient arrived in the OR at approximately 9:30 a.m. She was accompanied by two general surgeons, three plastic surgeons, two orthopedic surgeons and a state police detective who had been assigned to the patient. The detective informed me that she was there to take photographs of the patient's injuries.

The patient was lying supine on the stretcher. A cervical collar was being used to hold the dressing sponge that was covering a gaping wound on the left side of her mandible. Her face, hair, and body were caked in dried blood. Her entire body had sustained multiple stab wounds; some of the cuts were superficial and others were deep wounds. Her right elbow and left foot were covered with gauze sponges and wrapped with ace bandages. The patient also sustained a pneumothorax due to a stab wound to the right chest and had a large scalp laceration.

After the patient entered the OR, I asked the detective to remain in an area away from the sterile field while we readied the patient for surgery. I didn't have time to ask if she had been in an operating room setting before, but I had the impression that she hadn't. Somehow I sensed that she might have thought that we would leave the patient unattended on the OR table and that she would still need to be in charge. When she saw that the patient would not be left unattended, she relaxed somewhat.

The injuries sustained by this little girl were horrific. It was difficult to comprehend who could perform such a violent act. In the background I could hear the surgeons talking about the patient's injuries. They too were astounded at the extent of her injuries and planning what would need to be done to repair them.

I knew I had to take control of my emotions to help this little girl. Perioperative nursing care adheres to specified standards and policies and procedures. Despite the fact that this was an emergency and everything was happening at a frantic pace, creating and maintaining a culture of safety was everyone's goal. Prior to providing care for the patient, I communicated to the surgeons and anesthesiologists that we were proceeding without surgical or anesthesia consents. We all agreed to proceed. A "time out" was conducted prior to the start of the surgical procedures performed on this patient. Throughout the procedures, communication between all surgical team members was open and ongoing.

The anesthetic induction went smoothly. After the intravenous lines had been placed, the general surgeon asked me to insert the Foley catheter. Before inserting the Foley catheter, the state police detective asked the general surgeon to ascertain whether the patient had been sexually assaulted. She had not. I then proceed to insert the Foley catheter.

After the patient had been anesthetized we began to remove her bandages. It was only then I saw the extent of her injuries. The skin on her right elbow had been de-gloved and the bone was exposed. The bandages on her left foot were removed. One of the surgeons described her foot injury as being "sliced by a guillotine." It appeared as if her big toe was being held in place by a thread.

For several hours I was the only circulating nurse. I was confronted with responsibilities that would best be handled by two or three circulating nurses. Using the nursing process and integrating critical thinking skills, I was able to demonstrate a systematic and organized approach in the overall patient care management of this trauma patient. Working in a collaborative manner with ancillary personnel allowed me to divide tasks between the two nursing assistants helping me care for this patient. Indirectly they contributed to the care of this patient in a professional manner.

What made the care of this patient different from other patients I have cared for during an emergency can be defined in one word—violence. Following the surgery, as I reflected on the day I couldn't help but feel shaken as I thought about the injuries this patient sustained. Visions of her injuries kept me from sleeping at night. Caring for this patient made me aware of my own vulnerability and how quickly life can change.

The final step in the nursing process is the evaluation and the outcome of the nursing care that we delivered. During a scheduled dressing change performed several days after the surgery, I met the patient's father for the first time. I told him I was with his daughter when she was brought to the operating room. Next I re-introduced myself to the patient while checking her hospital identification bracelet. The father bent over and softly whispered into his daughter's ear, "This is one of the nurses who took care of you when you arrived in the operating room." It was good for me to meet this patient once again under different circumstances. I was able to see how her body was beginning to restore itself, how her wounds were healing.

I was reminded of what the essence of nursing means to me. What constitutes the essence of nursing varies from one individual to another. For me, it is a blend of knowledge, skill, compassion, caring, human touch, and presence. Providing perioperative nursing care for all pediatric patients in a high-technology environment requires all of the above, including vigilance. Vigilance is about continually scanning activities in the room to make certain that the values of nursing actions are appropriate and taking steps to alleviate problems. Though I didn't have a patient care plan written down, intuitively I knew what to do.

Everyone who participated in the care of this patient was exceptional. There were no egos. The goal was to deliver safe and quality patient care, and that's exactly what we did. By working together as a team, I believe we created a place of healing. I am in awe of the extraordinary way everyone came together to ensure the patient's journey throughout the perioperative experience. Her postoperative outcome appeared to be favorable. And in the end I was reminded of the goodness that life has to offer.

Practicing a Patient-Focused Model

Marsha Babb, RN, BSN, MS, CNOR
Newark, Delaware

The perioperative patient-focused model is the conceptual framework used in perioperative nursing practice. As a whole, it illustrates the dynamic nature of the perioperative patient and family experience and the nursing presence throughout the care process. The model puts the emphasis on relationships and effective working partnerships that nurses build and maintain to meet the unique needs of our patients, their families, and other nurses and health care professionals. It reaches into the overall health of the communities in which we live. This story recounts a poignant experience I shared with a patient and his family—an experience that not only illustrates the patient-focused model, but also shows the powerful role perioperative nurses play in shaping the surgical experience for patients and their families.

My friend Otalie and I were returning from church on a dark, cold, rainy November morning when three cars slammed into the back of her car. Having no injuries ourselves, we hurried to check on the people in the other cars. After assessing them, we called three ambulances to rescue those trapped in their cars. As the ambulances arrived and those injured were being cared for, my friend and I stayed at the scene to give our statement to police and to offer assistance if needed. Several bystanders who lived in a nearby housing development walked up to the scene and asked us what had happened. One of these bystanders was a rather fragile looking man, about 56 years old and his skin had a yellow tint. Before he spoke, I realized that he wasn't well. We began talking about the accident, and I mentioned I was a perioperative nurse. After Mr. Brown (fictitious name) learned where I worked, he fired off several questions. "Do you work in heart surgery? Do you know Dr. L (fictitious name)? I'm having surgery on an aneurysm. It's pretty big. I had surgery on it a few years ago, and it's back." As he explained his condition, and I continued to assess his physical appearance, my heart sank. He's a redo aneurysm. These patients face many risks in surgery, and some do not survive.

We continued to talk for some time. When the ambulances pulled away and Otalie and I were about to leave, I put out my hand to Mr. Brown to say good bye and wish him well. "I want you to be my nurse," he said, rather suddenly. I did a double take. "Me?" This was not at all what I expected. He explained that he had been struggling with the decision to have surgery and he needed a friendly face in the operating room. Of course I would be there.

"Mr. Brown, I'll find your surgical date and I will be your nurse," I said, searching his eyes for acknowledgement. He made no reply. He hugged me, and we parted ways.

When I arrived at work the next morning, I checked

the schedule and found his name. I made sure that I was
circulating and on-call the day of his surgery. It would be
a difficult case. These patients often don't do well after
surgery because of co-morbidities. Prior to the surgery
I had an opportunity to read his history. Mr. Brown had
struggled for the last three months trying to decide whether
to have surgery or not. Because of the relentless depression
he experienced as he made this decision, he had been
moved through our schedule. He was forced to make an
impossible decision. Should he sit on the "time-bomb" in
his chest or run the odds with surgery. Odds were definitely
not in his favor.

With my stomach in my throat, I thought out loud,
"Mr. Brown can't live like this much longer. He might not ·
survive surgery either."

On the day of his surgery the admitting staff prepared
Mr. Brown for surgery. I checked him in and when the
team was ready, I wheeled Mr. Brown into the operating
room. He wasn't smiling, but he seemed to calm down
with a touch of my hand. We moved him to the OR bed
and the anesthesia care provider began a rapid induction.
"Mr. Brown," I said, touching his shoulder gently, "I'm
here for you, and I'm not leaving this room until you do."
He squeezed my hand tightly and looked into my eyes as I
whispered, "Mr.Brown, I'm here for you." His eyes closed
gently, and he was asleep.

As surgery got under way, Dr. L was able to repair the
aneurysm in the aortic arch very quickly, but as he finished
the ascending portion of the aorta, the descending aorta
began to enlarge quickly down into the abdomen. Above
the iliac arteries, the aneurysm grew to about 15 inches in
diameter. I watched as Dr. L was deciding what should be

done. He did the best that he could to repair the descending aneurysm. Over the course of 12 hours, Mr. Brown lost many units of blood and Dr. L was still operating. This was a complication that would not be remedied. Around 3 a.m. Mr. Browns's heart went into an agonal rhythm. My heart sank, realizing that I would be responsible for speaking with the family. He passed away at about 4 a.m.

With tears streaming down my cheeks, I prepared his body for viewing. I pushed the stretcher through the doorway into the holding area and sent for the family. The OR doors opened and the family filed in around the stretcher. It took several moments for them to take in what they were seeing as Mr. Brown's body lay there motionless on the stretcher. Mr. Brown's wife, grown children, and a brother were present and they moved close to the stretcher to stroke his hand.

I spoke to the wife first, searching for words. "I am so sorry for your loss," I said, forcing myself to appear calm. "I met Mr. Brown a few weeks ago near your home. I told him I would be there for him, that I would be his nurse." His wife struggled to choke back her tears and his brother said, "You're the one he told us about." "You know who I am?" I asked. Mr Brown's brother said, "Yes, he said that he would have a friend in the OR, the last face he would see, and it would be you, his nurse, Marsha." My heart was racing as I moved toward Mrs. Brown. "How wonderful to know that you were there to comfort him just like you promised," said Mrs. Brown, sobbing. With my heart in my throat, I held out my arms to comfort them. They responded with hugs and tears.

With a patient-focused approach, there is an ongoing process to seek out and determine what is important to the person and family receiving care. This approach adopts the perspective of the person and family. This complex challenge requires an emphasis on relationships and building effective working partnerships with our patients and families. Mr. Brown had chosen me, and I had promised. For perioperative nurses, this is the cornerstone of our relationships with our patients and families. To me this is the heart of the OR.

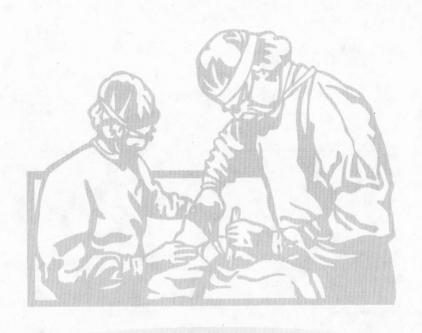